G000155205

Eat Yourself Thin

Copyright © 2006 Christine A. Dowse
All rights reserved.
ISBN: 1-4196-4639-7

To order additional copies, please contact us.
BookSurge, LLC
www.booksurge.com
1-866-308-6235
orders@booksurge.com

CHRISTINE A.
DOWSE

EAT YOURSELF
THIN

2006

Eat Yourself Thin

CONTENTS

***

INTRODUCTION

I discovered this way of eating when I found out I had gallstones. I didn't want invasive surgery, so I looked at natural ways to keep them from playing up. Because I had to change the way I ate, it also affected my husband, as he had to eat the same food. So by default he has lost weight too. I went from 16 ½ stone/*231 pounds** down to 10 stone/*147 pounds** in less than a year, this was from a dress size *22/16** down to my usual size *14/12/8**. My husband lost 2 stone/*28 pounds** and is now at his natural weight.

Before devising this eating plan, and because I was overweight, I found that my hips, knees, and ankles were painful, even after doing normal household tasks. I had no energy, and I couldn't walk very far without becoming breathless. Every day was like wading through thick treacle and everything was an effort. I was tired all the time and had no enthusiasm for life.

I couldn't wear the clothes I wanted to, as I felt I looked stupid in fashion clothes. All of my clothes, to me, looked like tents. I wouldn't look at myself in the mirror, as I didn't see the real me, only a person who was supposed to be me. I looked fat.

Because of the extra weight I couldn't wear high heels; if I did, I had to make sure I hadn't far to walk and was sitting down most of the time, because they made my feet ache and pulled on my back. My shoe size had also gone up by 2 sizes, as my feet had become fat as well.

Being overweight does affect every aspect of your life, including trying to fit in an aircraft seat, and I wanted my old self-back. Every aspect of my life had changed. I had been an energetic, zest for life person, a person who enjoyed meeting other people and going out. I had become a person who didn't want to go out, with no energy and no interest in life.

You may put a brave face and say you are happy and it doesn't bother you. The only person you are kidding is yourself. Everyone else tries to treat you normally, but they are mindful of what you can do and can't do; they must accommodate your inabilities and adjust their social lives to save you from embarrassment, e.g. like going swimming.

This eating plan is not just for an individual, it is for all the family. So you don't have to prepare meals just for yourself and other meals for the rest of the family, you can all eat the same. You can also use the recipes for dinner parties.

Age doesn't matter either. This plan is good for children as well as the elderly. It covers the whole spectrum of ages, and all ages will benefit.

Following this plan, we found our energy levels increased, which in turn meant we became more active; the tiredness left us. Because we had more energy and became more active it helped the weight go quicker. We found our memory recall became sharper, we didn't have to think so hard about things, and we just got on with it naturally.

You will find that your whole well-being improves. Your skin texture improves and becomes smooth and silky. The tiredness goes, you aren't so snappy or frustrated, you don't catch all of those bugs and infections flying around at work, your eyes sparkle again and you get back your zest for life. I am now living life again, having fun buying new clothes and twirling in front of the mirror in the changing rooms.

*USA

***

CHAPTER ONE
EATING PLAN VERSUS DIET

Everyone through life has tried to lose weight by dieting. Your success is achieved, the weight drops off you. Then you start to eat the odd snack, a packet of crisps/*chips**, all the things you previously cut back on, and the weight begins to go back on.

You can't keep on that diet forever, because you feel hungry all the time and are fed up of eating carrots in between meals. It has become bland and boring. The only trouble is, once you stop the diet the weight goes back on, plus some extra. So now you are bigger than before you started the diet.

You don't have to diet to lose weight. You don't have to join a gym to lose weight. You don't have to be on faddy diets to lose weight. You don't have to starve yourself to lose weight.

Losing weight is a matter of what you eat and how much—yes, how much. This is as much as you like; as long as you are sensible with the portions and you are not gluttonous. Stick to three meals a day, breakfast, lunch/dinner, dinner/tea and you can have one of the snacks for supper. You can have as much fruit and vegetables as you like, with meals or throughout the day. You will not feel hungry between meals. In fact you will naturally cut down on your intake of food, as that starving, hungry feeling goes.

On this eating plan, your body will take itself back to its own natural weight. In other words what you should be, what your body wants to be, where it feels right and right for you.

At first your body has to tone up from the inside; then it will take care of how your body looks outside. If the inside is not in tiptop condition, your body hasn't got the resources to care about the outer shell; it is taking all of its energy just surviving and keeping going. All of a sudden you will notice the changes, as will others, and the first sign usually, is in the face. It begins to glow and radiate, the eyes twinkle. The skin looks and feels smoother.

If you have a petrol driven car and fill it, by mistake, with diesel, it stops. The body is the same: Feed it and service it right, and it will be more efficient and run smoothly.

The body craves food for energy. If you eat the wrong foods, your body's metabolism is not being fed; this in turn makes your body store fat, as you are starving your body of vital nutrients and the body has gone into survival mode. Fat is a bit like keeping food in the cupboard, so you always have food at hand to eat. Starve your body of its vital nutrients and it will store fat, and you will want to eat more, as your body is telling you it is starving, when it really is not. It is trying to tell you that it needs the right food to survive. The body is like soil: If you do not fertilise the soil it will not produce good crops.

The body needs and requires a constant intake of nutrients; by starving the body of these essential elements you make yourself susceptible to ailments, illness and obesity. By feeding the body with junk food, and foods that are high in chemicals and additives, the body's defence mechanisms kick in, as they regard these things to be the enemy that is going to harm the body. Because your body is now getting the nutrients it requires, on the eating plan, you eat less. This is because your stomach shrinks, as it is not being overloaded and stretched with junk food.

You are responsible for your own well-being, no one else. You take care of everyone else in life and everything else in life, so why not yourself? If you don't pay the gas bill, they come and cut you off, so you make sure you pay it. So why do you neglect yourself, why are you torturing your body, why are you starving yourself to death? Take responsibility for yourself and don't be side tracked by all the bad foods, don't be tempted to eat these banned foods; the only person you are harming is yourself.

I have found this way of eating also helps people with attention seeking disorders, high blood pressure, heart problems, cholesterol, IBS, candida, gall stones, asthma and thyroid problems. I have had my friends on the eating plan to see if it does work for other people, and discovered it helped with their other ailments. All lost weight, gained energy and were less tired and their other symptoms were in decline. I put this down to the fact that all of the foods eaten had no chemicals, preservatives, or additives. This has led me to wonder how many more ailments and illnesses are attributed to these adulterated foods, and whether some of the illnesses would not happen if we all ate unadulterated food.

You will find, once you are in the habit of eating correctly and sneak a crisp/*chip** or two, that it will leave a funny taste in your mouth as if there were a plastic coating in your mouth. You can eventually eat some of the banned foods occasionally, but when you do, and especially if they have a high fat, chemical, additive or preservative content, your trips to the loo/*bathroom** will increase and your motions will be very loose—that is, if you can finish the food, as the taste in your mouth is awful and you won't enjoy it. The foods you used to favour, go out of favour, and you will begin to favour your new foods and the ideas of how to prepare your food.

You will learn to listen to your body, and can start off by looking at food, and asking your body if it wants it. The body's reaction is either *yuck* or *mmm*. This might sound a little stupid, but if you think about it, how many times have you said "I really fancy….", or take pregnant women—don't they fancy food? Often that fancying is the body's way of telling you that it is short in the nutrients that that food you want contains? This does not apply to anyone who has not started this eating plan, as their minds still rule their eating habits and their minds have not been trained to recognise good foods, nor have their bodies been retrained. It is like all bad habits: They are easy to pick up but harder to discard.

*USA

***

DON'T USE WEIGHING SCALES

NEVER use weighing scales, as your body's weight fluctuates with how you are feeling, what you are doing and, for women in particular, the time of the month.

You will judge your weight loss by your clothes, their tightness, and looseness. Weighing scales are banned, as they make you paranoid about not losing enough weight each day or week.

*****

EATING WELL DOESN'T HAVE TO BE TIME-CONSUMING OR EXPENSIVE

I know people lead busy lives, they always have. I haven't the time either to spend hours in the kitchen, nor have I loads of money for expensive foods or ingredients. But to eat well doesn't have to be expensive, tasteless, or time consuming, as you will see.

We have been led to believe it is faster to buy a ready meal, than cook your self a meal. It doesn't take very long to prepare and cook a good wholesome meal.

The couscous recipes (see recipes) take no more than half an hour from starting preparation to eating. Some dishes do take longer in preparation, but the cooking takes no longer than half an hour, if it is made on the top of the stove. If it is an oven dish, you can get on with something else, whilst it is cooking, or prepare and cook the night before and reheat the next day.

Cooking your food from scratch gives you a sense of satisfaction that you have created this masterpiece, and you know what you are eating.

Healthy food is cooked simply and quickly. The taste should come from the food itself, not fancy sauces, salt and sugar, which often mask tasteless food.

If you use organic produce, you will find it does not require as much cooking time as chemically produced food. With organic vegetables, you will discover a taste that does not exist with chemically grown vegetables. Organically grown vegetables taste as nature intended the vegetable to taste, and contains the nutrients that chemically produced food does not.

You will see from the part telling you about sugar, salt, water and hydrogenated fat, why cooking your own meals, from fresh ingredients, is important for your health and weight.

Not only will you improve your health but also your wealth. The weight in your purse/*wallet** will get heavier, but your body weight goes down, you will be amazed how much money you will save by cooking your own meals.

*USA

***

WHY YOU SHOULDN'T EAT IT

The main rule is to say to your self, "I AM ALLERGIC TO FAT, CHEMICALS, PRESERVATIVES AND ADDITIVES. I AM NOT DESIGNED TO EAT THESE". Just imagine that by eating too much of these foods you will be dead in a week.

Just imagine in 2,000 years time, an archaeologist unearthed your remains, and you were perfectly preserved. He/she would look at you and say, "Oh, this one ate too many foods containing preservatives. All this person did was kill themselves and preserve the body for us to find. Thank goodness common sense ruled eventually and preservatives were banned in food, otherwise we might have ended up the same".

Try as much as you can to eat organic and home-cooked food. By going back to basics and cooking your food yourself, you know exactly what you are eating. You will notice a difference if you go out to eat. The taste will not be very nice; you will be able to pick up the taste of excessive salt, sugar, fats, chemicals, and preservatives. This is because your taste buds have been re-educated to good wholesome food. The other thing you will notice, when you go out to eat, once you begin the eating plan, is loose faeces when you go to the toilet/*bathroom**. This will be due to the high fat content, etc., of the food. If you become constipated it is due to the high salt content and lack of fresh vegetables/fruit. I find I am more particular about where I choose to eat out, as the choice of fresh food is limited; most places, to keep costs down, go for catering packs of ready-made, ready to heat, and packeted foods.

*USA

***

WATER

If you live in an area where the water has been fluoridated, filter all water for boiling in the kettle or cooking. Drink only bottled water, as this has only the natural level of fluoride content in the water. Also, do not use toothpaste containing fluoride. By using this type of toothpaste, you are overloading your system with fluoride. It has been known since 1854 that excessive fluoride inhibits the thyroid gland function. This means that your thyroid function is thrown out of kilter. The thyroid governs your metabolic rate and, it produces the iodine for the body to function. Mainly it makes the thyroid function under-active, leaving you feeling lethargic, tired, out of breath, and putting on weight, to name but a few. In most instances by eliminating fluoridated water and fluoride toothpaste, can, in some cases, restore your thyroid function to normal.

***

SUGAR AND SALT

Because so many foods contain excessive sugar and salt, our bodies become reliant on high sugar intake for that energy boost. The trouble is that most of that intake turns to fat and makes you go up in energy, and a few hours later back down. So it becomes a vicious cycle of your body saying it needs that quick fix.

You need to feed the body with natural sugars. These come in the form of fruit and honey. When you do need a fix, turn to fruit, pure fruit juice, or honey. One good way is to make a fruit smoothie (see recipes). You can make these up to take to work (see ideas for snacks).

Glucose occurs naturally in fruits and vegetables and a number of other foods. These natural sugars are easily absorbed and used by the body. Glucose is always present in our bloodstream and is essential for metabolic functions.

Sucrose or refined sugar; is so refined, it has no nutritional value whatsoever and is of no value to the body. Refined sugars give a rush of energy, by making a massive secretion of insulin, the hormone responsible for regulating blood sugar levels and storing fat. This is why you are high one minute and then low. You keep feeding your body this way, and your mood swings are great and the fat goes on. This can lead to diabetes. Sucrose also damages our healthy cells by robbing them of electrons, and eventually the cell dies.

By limiting your sugar intake to small amounts, you can also slow down the aging process. Sugar becomes blood sugar and bonds with the proteins in your body's tissue, and the indications are grey hair and premature aging. Sugar intake has also been linked to cancer, Parkinson's and Alzheimer's disease. Complete removal of sugar from the diet has seen reductions and recoveries from cancer, diabetes, and heart disease.

You cannot eliminate refined sugar completely from your diet, as sometimes there is no other substitute you can use; e.g. in stewed fruit and jam, as you would have to use an inordinate amount of honey to sweeten apples, rhubarb or jam, if you are making large quantities.

***

SALT

Salt makes you thirsty; you then drink more, often the wrong type of liquid. Even if you just drink water, the salt has to be washed out of your system, because the body becomes dehydrated, from the intake of too much salt. Most ready-made foods and sauces have too much salt in them. They are put in to make these foods tasty, as is sugar. Crisps/*chips**

are a good example of salty food; they are coated in salt and chemical flavourings. If someone gave you two bowls, one filled with the equivalent amount of salt and the other with the flavouring substance, as in a packet of crisps, and said, eat those bowls of salt and flavouring substances, you would say no, and even if you did eat it, you would soon feel sick.

Use sea salt and freshly milled pepper to season your food.

*USA

***

HYDROGENATED FAT
This fat is commonly known as Trans fat, and it dangerous to your health. It can contribute to inflamed and it stiffens arteries, raise LDL (bad cholesterol), lower HDL (good cholesterol), diabetes, heart disease, you can put excessive weight on, around the abdomen, even if you are on a diet, as some of the diet products contain trans fats.

Trans fats occur naturally in small amounts in food, mostly in meat and dairy products, these are not harmful, as they are naturally occurring.

Trans fats that are harmful are the artificial ones found in some processed foods, commercially manufactured biscuits, cakes and pastry, margarine, some snack bars and sweets, powdered drinks and products used to enhance drinks.

Hydrogenated fat/oil is made by heating vegetable oil or fat to a very high temperature, then hydrogen is "bubbled" through it, creating a chemical reaction and the end result is a substance similar to plastic. Commercial producers of food like to use hydrogenated fat in their products, as it gives the products a longer shelf life, and is cheap to use. Trans fats are by-products of the hydrogenation process.

Any foods that state on their labels, "Contains Hydrogenated fats or oils", will also contain trans fats. If the hydrogenated fat/oil comes near the top of the list of ingredients on an item of food, the more trans fats there are in the product.

On a list of ingredients, "contained in the food", the first item has the highest content presence in that food, the second lower than the first and so on. So the last item on the list has the least content presence in the product.

***

CHAPTER TWO
DETOXIFICATION

FIRST STAGE

The first step is to detoxify the body. But don't worry it is not painful and you won't be going hungry. But you must be ready to ditch all fast foods, foods with chemicals, preservatives and additives, which means reading labels on food, including what you think is good food. Listed below is a list of banned foods.

During the first few weeks, we have to detoxify your body. Detoxifying the body is important, as all the waste is eliminated from the body that has built up over the years of neglect, by not eating correctly. By drinking the apple juice, water and following the eating plan, and following the dietary suggestions that follow, the detoxification is painless and will not harm the body. This enables the body to eat up the fat that is stored in the body, and to start the change we have to flush the system out. This is not a painful process, and you can still eat; it is a case of getting the body to do what it is meant to do naturally. Because of all the processed foods and chemicals ingested in the body through time, the body becomes clogged and forgets how to rid itself of unwanted waste.

To start with, drink at least a litre of pure apple juice every day. This is the biggest key to detoxifying the body. Keep on with the apple juice all the time. You do not have to forgo your tea or coffee, just be sensible; you can drink as much bottled water, as you want. As for alcohol, you will have to limit this to one or two glasses a week, as the sugar content does not help the system. You can up the amount later on, but it would be beneficial for the body if you don't go mad. Binge drinking is definitely out. One of the best ways if you go out with your mates for a drink, is to have one alcoholic drink and one large glass of water alternately. This way you won't have a hangover in the mornings and you won't drink as much, nor will you feel an odd ball in the group.

During this time you may experience a lot of visits to the loo/*bathroom**, so stock up on the toilet paper and air freshener! As the body detoxifies, and you are following the eating plan, you will find that your motions should not be as odorous. This lack of strong odour is a good indicator that your body is functioning well, if you eat the wrong food, for any reason, your motions will have a strong odour.

Your energy levels will begin to rise, and you will feel more alert, the weight loss will occur slowly after two to three weeks. Losing weight should not be fast. It is better to lose a few pounds a week; this way the body readjusts and the weight stays off, providing you keep on eating correctly and don't start eating junk food.

To start this eating plan, here are the foods that you cannot eat. We will discuss some of the banned foods later on.

*USA

BANNED FOODS
Any ready meals
Ready sauces or ready mix sauces
Processed foods
Burgers
Fish and chips
Chips/*fries**
Indian and Chinese take away
Pizzas
Kebabs
Cheese
Butter
Cream
Any fat
Biscuits/*cookies** – shop bought
Cakes – shop bought

Pastry
Crisps/*chips**
Fizzy drinks/carbonated drinks
Squash/*cordial** drinks
Tin soup
Frozen processed food
Pre-packed sandwich meat
Sweeteners
Gravy granules
Full fat milk
Fancy breakfast cereal
Ice-lolly pops
Ice cream
Sweets
Chocolate
Mayonnaise
Water with added flavourings
Tinned sausages
Check tinned/*canned** vegetables and fruit for added salt and sugar

*USA

YOU CAN SUBSTITUTE THE BANNED FOODS WITH

Stock cubes
Low fat cheese – only once a week
Parmesan cheese
Low fat spread
Light mayonnaise
Cooked meat from the deli counter
Cereal bars – no more than 2 a day
Plain cereals – not novelty ones
Porridge

FOODS THAT HAVE NO LIMITS

Meat
Fish
Eggs

Vegetables, including potatoes
Fruit
Dried fruit
Pasta
Rice
Herbs

***

ONE THIRD RULE

Once you have started on the eating plan you will find that your body does not crave food. The secret is that if you feed the body properly, it will only want to be fed at the correct time, i.e. when it is mealtime. You must eat regularly: breakfast, lunch/dinner, dinner/tea. Do not leave the table hungry, listen to your body. A correctly fed body is a happy body.

At each mealtime you must remember the one-third rule. Each dinner plate must have one-third protein (meat, fish, eggs etc), just over one third vegetable, and just under one third carbohydrates (potatoes, rice, pasta, etc.). In your sandwiches, it is the same: The bread counts as the carbohydrate, then the meat/fish, then the salad or other vegetables or fruit. You must keep this balance for these two meals, lunch and dinner, because this way you will feel full until the next meal. For vegetarians, use products that are equivalent to meat, fish etc.

You can still have your roast dinners and gravy, just remember to use oil and not animal fat for the roast potatoes. You can still have your steaks and chops. Just remember the one-third rule.

If you have your main meal at night, try not to eat later than 7 pm. After the usual tidying up process that a mealtime creates, try to take a brisk walk or do some gardening; this helps the digestive action to begin, and will help with the flatulence problem. If you just flop in a chair the meal lies heavy in your stomach, and your body has no use for the meal you have just given it. As you are not sending any signals for energy, the body then stores this food as it is, and then turns it into fat for when the energy is needed. This only applies to main meal of the day. If you ate at midday, you would be naturally active throughout the afternoon, burning off the intake of food.

***

WATCH FOR CHEMICAL ADDITIVES, AND EAT LOCALLY SOURCED FOOD

Check all chemical additives in any food you buy, as it is these that inhibit the body in losing weight. The chemical residues build up in the body, damaging the immune system so that it cannot fight illnesses and viruses effectively. This also stops the body taking the vital nutrients from the food you are about to eat.

Try to eat locally sourced food. This helps the body to build up the immune system, as you are eating food grown and raised in the environment where you live. This food has been taking in all of the germs, pollutants, etc., particular to your environment. Then when you visit other areas of the country or world, your body's immune system has enough energy to combat "foreign" bugs and germs, until the body adjusts to the new environment, by eating food of that locality. The body can recognise differences, it then adds those immunities to its bank of fighters.

Also, locally grown, raised, and seasonal foods are fresher than those that have travelled for miles. This travelling causes the produce to deteriorate in transit, and the nutritional values drop. So have a good percentage of local produce to combat the nutritional loss of the not-so-local produce.

Some people say they have (and some do have) a wheat allergy. Most of the time it is the chemicals the wheat has been sprayed with, and in shop-bought bread it is the additives that are affecting the body, not the wheat.

Even the good old loaf of bread is now full of additives and preservatives. Do you suffer from flatulence and feel bloated after eating bread? It is your body's way of trying to get rid of the bad things, and it is your body that swells up when something is not right, especially the stomach area. The easiest way to explain this is to take the common pimple. The body's defence mechanism is to fight it, and the white corpuscles surrounding the offending matter, it swells up with pus and you get rid of it. The same happens in the stomach, hence bloating, and wind.

I would recommend a bread-making machine, so you can make your own bread, and you know there are no additives or preservatives in it. Also you won't need to eat as much of homemade bread because it is denser and not full of air. Once you have tasted it you will never look back. Also this bread is not fattening as you can make it with olive oil and honey. There are recipes for bread in the book.

***

CHAPTER THREE
IDEAS FOR MEALS

Breakfast/ lunch or tea

Tinned fruit, with the juice strained off – half a tin is usually enough for one person, two dessert spoons of low fat natural yoghurt spooned over the top of the fruit, one teaspoon of runny honey drizzled over the yoghurt. After a while, when the taste buds have adjusted, you will not necessarily need the honey, or as much honey.

Porridge made with semi skimmed milk – half a cup of oats, one and a quarter cups of milk. Place in a deep bowl and microwave for 4 ½ minutes, stirring half way through. Leave to cool for two mins and drizzle one teaspoon of honey over the top to sweeten.

Homemade bread toasted. No more than 3 slices of bread. Spread thinly with a low fat spread. You can use jam, but make sure it is organic jam or marmalade, or honey, spread thinly.

Fruit smoothies (see recipes).

Low fat yoghurt

Plain cereal with chopped organic banana and or sultanas on the top – the banana and sultanas will replace the honey, or any chopped or sliced fresh fruit.

Soup (see recipes).

Pancakes with sweet or savoury filling (see recipes).

Homemade bread sandwiches.

Jacket potato with Winter Salad.

Winter Salad with tinned mackerel in tomato sauce.

You can have as much fruit juice as you like; it must be pure fruit juice, and do not have orange or grapefruit, as it is too acidic.

To sweeten use honey, remember that honey sweetens more than sugar, so if you had two spoons of sugar you would only need a level teaspoon or less of honey. Do not use other sweeteners.

Try to drink tea in the morning with your breakfast and after every meal, as it aids the digestive system.

Combination ideas
Pure fruit juice, homemade bread toasted with jam or honey.
Pure fruit juice, cereal with fruit.
Low fat yoghurt, homemade bread toasted with jam or honey.
Tea with no milk, so make it weak tea if you usually have milk.
Coffee with no milk, again make it weak if you usually take milk.

You can use your own recipes, but do make sure there is no fat used in the preparation. You will get the entire natural fat you need from meat or fish to benefit the body.

***

IDEAS FOR
Lunch/Dinner
Choose one of these main courses:
Oven baked beans
Lamb Rissoles
Beef Rissoles
Couscous with Salmon
Couscous with Smoked Bacon
Tagliatelle and Chorizo

<u>Combine with one of these vegetables with meat, fish, or eggs, for vegetarians use equivalent protein substitute.</u>
Winter Salad
Nutmeg Carrots
Candy Floss Leeks
Spinach with low-fat Cream Cheese or Feta Cheese
Chunky Chopped Roast Veg
Creamy Mashed Potatoes and variations
Aubergine Bake

<u>IDEAS FOR SWEETS</u>
Greek yoghurt drizzled with a teaspoon of honey.
Stewed fruit, with low fat natural yoghurt.
Strawberries/raspberries, with low fat natural yoghurt, drizzled with a teaspoon of honey.
Smoothies made thick.
Bananas and custard.
Any fruit.

***

CHAPTER FOUR
RECIPES

I hope you have fun rediscovering food and learn how to enjoy the taste of real food again. Experiment with your own recipes, remembering to substitute any fat or cream content with the alternatives.

SMOOTHIES

STRAWBERRY SMOOTHIE
1 avocado peeled and sliced off the stone
8 oz/225g strawberries
3 dessert spoons of low fat natural yoghurt
1 dessert spoon honey
Half a cup of either pure mango juice, apple juice or pineapple juice.

METHOD
Place all the ingredients, roughly chopped, in a blender and blitz.

MANGO SMOOTHIE
1 banana
1 mango
3 dessertspoons of low fat yoghurt
2 tsp honey
Half a cup of either pure mango juice or pineapple juice

METHOD
Place all the ingredients, roughly chopped, in a blender and blitz.
The less juice you put in, the thicker the smoothie, and you can eat it like yoghurt.

***

PANCAKES WITH SWEET AND SAVOURY FILLINGS

BATTER MIX
4 oz/110 g self-raising flour/flour plus half tsp baking powder*.
1 egg.
4 tablespoons of semi skimmed milk.
Water.

METHOD
Put flour in a bowl.
Break in the egg and add the milk.
Mix to a semi stiff paste, if too stiff add a little more milk.
Gradually add the water, mixing all the time, until the consistency of thick cream.
Heat a large non-stick frying pan.
Put one ladle of the batter mixture into a very hot pan and swish around the pan, so it covers the base of the pan.
Turn over when cooked on the underside.
Place in a warm oven, on a plate, when cooked.
Repeat until all of the mixture is used.

Take one pancake at a time and fill with the desired filling.

FILLINGS

STEWED APPLES
2 large cooking apples
3 tbsp honey
4 fluid oz/120 ml water
Light natural yoghurt
Honey for garnish

METHOD
Peel and core the apples, then slice the apple into chunks.
Put the water into a medium sized pan.
Add apples and honey.
Cook over a moderate heat until nearly boiling; turn down the heat and

simmer until the apples are soft. Some will turn to mush; be sure to stir at regular intervals.

Depending on the apples, it will take about 10 to 15 minutes to cook.

Place filling in a pancake and fold in half, then half again, or roll into a tube.

Put some light natural yoghurt over the top and drizzle with 1 tsp of honey.

The stewed apple is also good on its own with natural yoghurt spooned over the top.

You can also use fresh rhubarb, apricots, or any suitable fresh fruit.

*USA

SAVOURY FILLINGS

TUNA
1 small tin of tuna in brine
2 tbsp light mayonnaise
2 tbsp frozen sweet corn or 2 large chopped fresh tomatoes

METHOD
Mix the tuna and mayonnaise in a bowl.
Add the sweet corn or tomatoes.
Microwave on high for 1 ½ to 2 minutes, depending on the wattage of your microwave.

MUSHROOM SAUCE
4 medium mushrooms, sliced
¼ pint/150 ml semi skimmed milk
1 oz/25 g of butter
Salt and pepper to taste
2 heaped tsp cornflour

METHOD

Place all the ingredients in a pan and season with salt and pepper.
Bring nearly to the boil and simmer for 15 minutes.
Mix the cornflour down with a little water until it is liquid.
Pour the cornflour into the pan, stirring all the time, until the mixture thickens.

To make up
Put some of the tuna mix into a pancake and roll up into a tube.
Fill the other pancakes, place three on a plate, this amount is for you main meal of the day, for breakfast or lunch make one or two pancake rolls, and pour over some of the mushroom sauce on each plate.
Serve.

You can use tinned salmon, mackerel in tomato sauce or any other filling you would like.

For vegetarians, omit the fish and use both tomatoes and sweet corn.

***

BREAD RECIPIES

BASIC BREAD RECIPIE
10 fl oz/300 ml water
2 tbsp extra virgin olive oil
1 dessertspoon of honey
1lb/450 g white bread flour
1 ½ level tsp salt
1 sachet dried yeast

METHOD
Put the water, olive oil and honey in the bread maker container.
Add the flour and make a well either side of the paddle; in one well put the salt, and in the other well put the yeast.
Put in the breadmaker and follow appliance instructions.

VARIATIONS FOR BREAD
SESAME SEED AND SUNFLOWER SEED BREAD

Add 3 tbsp of sunflower seeds and 4 tbsp sesame seeds to the flour; mix carefully in the flour, before putting in the breadmaker.

WALNUT BREAD
Add 2 tbsp walnuts, more if you want, to the flour before mixing in as above.

DATE BREAD
Add 4oz/100 g of dates to the flour before mixing in as above.

SUN DRIED TOMATO AND PARMESAN CHEESE BREAD
Put water, extra virgin olive oil, honey, and 4 large (6 medium) chopped sun-dried tomatoes in the bread maker container.
Weigh the flour and add 4 tbsp of dried or fresh Parmesan cheese to the flour; mix into the flour.
Add to the other ingredients in the bread maker container as above.

SULTANA BREAD
Mix 4oz/110 g of sultanas to the flour, before mixing in as above.

You can make any variation you want as long as you remember to put all liquid ingredients in first and then the dry things.

All flour that is used for making bread must be bread flour.

BROWN BREAD
10 fl oz/300 ml water
2 tbsp extra virgin olive oil
1 dessertspoon treacle
10 oz/275 g brown bread flour
6 oz/175 g white bread flour
1 ½ level tsp salt
1 sachet dried yeast

METHOD
Put water, extra virgin olive oil and honey into the bread maker container.

Mix the two flours together.

Put the flour on top of the liquid ingredients.

Make a well either side of the paddle in the flour; in one well put the salt and in the other put the yeast.

Put in the breadmaker and follow the appliance instructions.

GRANARY BREAD

8oz/225 g of granary bread flour

4oz/110g brown flour

4oz/110g white flour

10floz/300 ml water

2 tbsp extra virgin olive oil

1 dessert spoon treacle

1 ½ level tsp salt

1 sachet dried yeast

METHOD

Mix all flours together, and then make up as for white bread.

BROWN BREAD WITH APRICOTS

10floz/300 ml water

2 tbsp extra virgin olive oil

1 dessert spoon treacle

8oz/225g brown bread flour

8oz/225g white bread flour

About 6 dried apricots, more if you want it depending on the size of them

1 ½ level tsp of salt

1 sachet dried yeast

METHOD

Put water, olive oil, and treacle in the bread maker container. Mix the flours and snipped up apricots together, put in the bread maker container. Add the salt and yeast as before.

You can use the apricots in the white bread as well.

***

SOUPS

POTATO AND PARSNIP CURRY SOUP
1 onion, finely chopped
1 ½ lb/700g of potatoes
10 oz/275g parsnips
1 tbsp curry powder
1 pint/550 ml vegetable stock
¼ pint/150 ml semi skimmed milk
To make creamier you can add ¼ inch/7 mm of block-creamed coconut.
Extra light olive oil
Salt

METHOD
In a large pan add the olive oil and fry onion until clear.
Dice peeled potatoes and parsnips and add to the onions in the pan.
Put in the curry powder and stir well, coating the vegetables.
Add stock, milk, and creamed coconut, if used.
Simmer for 20 minutes.
Take off the heat and leave to stand for 5 minutes, until it has cooled down a bit.
Season with a little salt.
Liquidise in a blender or food processor, and serve.

CARROT AND PARSNIP COCONUT SOUP
Extra light olive oil
1 onion, finely chopped
2 large parsnips, peeled and diced
3 large carrots, peeled and diced
2 pints/1.1L chicken stock
¼ inch/7 mm of block creamed coconut
Salt

METHOD

Heat oil in a large saucepan, add the onion, and cook until clear.

Add parsnips, carrots, stock, and creamed coconut; bring to the boil and stir occasionally whilst it is coming to the boil.

Simmer for 25 minutes.

Remove from the heat and let stand for 5 minutes.

Season with a little salt.

Liquidise in a blender or food processor and serve.

LEEK, CARROT AND LENTIL SOUP

2 medium leeks, peeled and finely sliced

4 large carrots, peeled and grated

6 oz/170 g red lentils

1 pint/550 ml fresh chicken stock

1 tbsp extra light olive oil

Salt and pepper

METHOD

Put oil into a large saucepan, over a moderate heat.

Sweat the leeks until soft in the saucepan.

Add grated carrots.

Add stock and lentils.

Season with salt and pepper.

Simmer for 30 to 45 minutes.

Leave to stand over night.

Reheat and serve.

***

MAIN DISHES

RECIPIES

You can mix and match these recipes for any mealtime.

OVEN BAKED BEANS

4oz/125 g dried butter beans (soaked overnight in cold water)
1 red onion, finely chopped
1 clove of garlic, finely chopped
1 tin of chopped tomatoes
Half a tsp of dried oregano
Quarter of a tsp of freshly grated nutmeg
Good pinch of dried coriander
Good pinch of dried cumin
1 dessert spoon of tomato puree
Salt and pepper
1 tbsp light olive oil

METHOD

Put butter beans in a large bowl and cover well with cold water; if the beans swell out of the water, add more cold water. They roughly treble in size when soaked. Leave for at least 12 hours to soak.

When beans are fully expanded drain in a colander.

Heat 1 tbsp of light olive oil in a frying pan.

Gently fry the onion, add the garlic, —don't burn.

Add tin tomatoes, oregano, coriander, cumin, tomato puree, salt and pepper, and stir well.

Take off the heat.

Place beans in a casserole dish, pour over the tomato mixture, and gently mix.

Put a lid on the casserole dish and place in the oven at 200 C/400 F/gas mark 6 for 45 minutes, turn down the heat to 150 C/300 F/gas mark 2 for a further 3 hours, and stir if necessary.

Turn off the oven and leave beans in the oven till cool.

This dish is best left to stand overnight and reheat.

The beans can be made well in advance. You can either keep them in the fridge in the casserole dish, or freeze in portions. You can microwave to warm through.

This dish is not eaten hot; it needs to be eaten just over warm.

LAMB RISSOLES

1lb/450g minced lamb
1 red onion
1 clove of garlic, finely chopped

Half a tsp dried oregano
Good pinch dried cumin
2 tsp freshly grated nutmeg
1 dessert spoon of tomato puree
Salt and pepper
Plain flour

METHOD

Place roughly chopped onion in a food processor and process until onion is finely chopped.

Add lamb, garlic, oregano, cumin, nutmeg, salt and pepper, tomato puree.

Blitz until it is a fine mixture.

Tip out onto a heavily floured board. Make into a long sausage. Divide into 8 equal pieces.

Pat each piece, one at a time, flat and fold so the flour is mixed in with the meat; pat and fold twice more.

Roll into sausage shape and place in an ovenproof dish.

When all pieces are in the dish, place in the oven at 200 C/400 F/gas mark 6 for approx 45 minutes, depending on the thickness of the lamb rissole and your oven.

When cooked, remove from the oven and leave to stand for about 5–7 minutes. Do not eat straight from the oven, as the meat needs to rest.

This dish goes well with oven-baked beans.

This recipe can be made a day in advance and stored in the fridge, before cooking, in a dish, covered with cling film. Remove the cling film before cooking.

BEEF RISSOLES

1lb/450g of minced beef
1 beef stock cube
1 red onion
1 clove of garlic
2 tbsp tomato puree
Good pinch of dried cumin

Salt and pepper
Plain flour

METHOD

Place roughly chopped onion in a food processor and blitz until finely chopped.

Add mince, crumbled beef stock, garlic, tomato puree, cumin, salt and pepper into the processor.

Blitz until it is a fine mixture.

Tip out onto a heavily floured board. Make into a long sausage and divide into equal sized pieces.

Take each piece and pat into a round of about three quarters of an inch/20 mm thick, so it is now a patty shape.

Place in an ovenproof dish.

Put in the oven at 200 C/400 F/gas mark 6 for 30 minutes to 45 minutes, or until the meat is cooked.

Remove from oven; leave to stand for 2–3 mins before serving.

COUSCOUS – 2-3 servings

4oz/110g couscous
6 fluid ounces/175 ml cold water
1 tbsp extra light olive oil
Salt and pepper to taste

METHOD

Put oil in a pan, add couscous, swish around, and add water.

Put a lid on the pan, place on a moderate heat to warm through. Do not bring to the boil. As the couscous begins to swell and soak up the water, stir with a fork. When all of the water has been absorbed, remove the pan from the heat to stand for at least 5 minutes, stirring occasionally. Add the salt and pepper and stir in. Leave the lid on the pan.

COUSCOUS WITH SALMON – complete meal

Make couscous as above.

1 tin of drained salmon, take out all of the bones and skin. Chop roughly.

OR
1 packet of smoked salmon bits.
1 onion, finely chopped.
A selection of vegetables cut into bite size pieces and cook in boiling water until they are *al dente.*
2 large mushrooms, optional.
1 tbsp extra light olive oil.
Salt and pepper

METHOD
Place a large frying pan onto a moderate to high heat.
Put extra light olive oil into the frying pan, when the pan is warm and fry the onion.
Add mushrooms, cook until just browning.
Turn off the heat.
Put the couscous back onto a low heat and add the salmon to the couscous; stir in.
Add the drained *al dente* vegetables to the couscous, and stir.
Add salt and pepper, stir with a fork and serve.

COUSCOUS WITH SMOKED BACON – complete meal
Make couscous as above.
6 rashers of smoked back bacon, trimmed of all fat, chop into chunks.
1 onion, finely diced.
1 clove of garlic, finely diced.
2 large mushrooms, thinly sliced.
Selection of vegetables, as above.
Salt and pepper.
1 tsp of extra light olive oil.

METHOD
Put light olive oil into a large frying pan, as above.
Fry chopped bacon and onion.
As the onion is turning clear add the garlic. Stir all the time to stop sticking.
Add the mushrooms – when the mushrooms are turning brown, add the vegetables and stir well.
Add salt and pepper to taste.
Stir the bacon mixture into the couscous and serve.

TAGLIATELLE AND CHORIZO- complete meal
4/5 balls tagliatelle
Half of a good chorizo with paprika, sliced thinly
1 tin of chopped tomatoes
1 onion, finely diced
3 large mushrooms, finely sliced
4 dessert spoons of grated Parmesan cheese
Salt and pepper
Light olive oil

METHOD
Put oil in a deep frying pan and fry onions until clear.
Add mushrooms and fry until tender but not brown.
Add chorizo and the tin tomatoes to the pan.
Add a little salt and pepper; you will not need much as the chorizo is spicy.
Stir in 2 dessertspoons of the Parmesan cheese.
Turn down the heat and simmer.
Cover the pan with a lid and leave to simmer for 20 minutes. Check half way through and give the mixture a stir.
At the same time prepare enough tagliatelle as per the instructions on the packet.
Drain the tagliatelle and place in portions on the plates, and then spoon the chorizo mix over the top. Divide the remaining Parmesan cheese and sprinkle over the chorizo mix.

***

VEGETABLES

WINTER SALAD
1 carrot
Red and white cabbage as needed
1 onion (optional)

METHOD

Using a Mandolin, finely slice enough red cabbage and white cabbage for your needs, also 1 carrot.

Thinly slice 4 slices of onion rings for garnish, if desired.

Mix the cabbages and carrot together in a bowl and serve, garnishing with the onion rings, which will have been separated.

This is a good accompaniment with jacket potatoes and meat dishes, or you can eat it on its own, for a change, instead of adding the onions, add sultanas in the mix.

You can use this as a base for tin mackerel in tomato sauce poured over the top as a meal or a snack.

NUTMEG CARROTS

2 large carrots
1 oz/25 g of butter
½ tsp of fresh grated nutmeg

METHOD

Finely slice carrots.

Put the butter in a pan.

Add carrots and grated fresh nutmeg on the top of the carrots.

Put lid on pan, place on medium heat. When the butter is just starting to melt, gently stir the carrots, nutmeg and butter, so incorporating all the ingredients. Shake carrots around to mix in the pan regularly.

Cook for about 5 mins.

Take off heat and leave to stand for 2-3 mins.

CANDY FLOSS LEAKS

1 leek, finely sliced
1 oz/25 g of butter

METHOD

Very finely slice leaks or chiffonade into thin strips.

Put the butter in the middle of the pan and place the leaks on top. Add a little salt.

Place over a medium heat until butter begins to melt, gently stir the leeks and butter, incorporating the ingredients.

Turn heat down to low.

Toss leaks in the pan to prevent burning.

Cook for 2-3 mins, or until the leeks are cooked as it will depend on how thick you have sliced the leeks.

SPINACH WITH LOW FAT CREAM CHEESE OR FETA CHEESE

1 bag of spinach
4-oz/110g low fat cream cheese

METHOD

Prepare and cook spinach, drain spinach and return to pan.

Add the chunks of cheese and fold in.

Serve at once.

Makes a complete meal or snack with a poached egg on top of the cooked spinach.

CHUNKY CHOPPED ROAST VEG

3 large carrots, peeled
3 large parsnips, peeled
1 large leek
8 mushrooms
6 large tomatoes
1 large courgette
1 large onion
4 cloves of garlic
Extra light olive oil
Salt and pepper to taste

METHOD

Prepare vegetables.

Chop all vegetables thickly and put in a large mixing bowl; pour over enough olive oil to thoroughly coat all vegetables, leaving some olive oil standing in the bottom of the bowl.

Leave to stand for 30 minutes to infuse the garlic and onion.

Place in a pre-heated oven 200 C/400 F/ gas mark 6, for approximately 30 minutes.

Serve straight away.

CREAMY MASHED POTATOES AND VARIATIONS
4 medium potatoes

METHOD
Boil potatoes, drain, and return to pan.

Add dash of milk, 2 oz/56g low fat spread, and salt and pepper.

Mash until smooth and creamy.

VARATIONS
Follow steps as above, but add after mashing:

1 dessertspoon grain mustard stirred in.

OR

Chives finely chopped and stirred in.

OR

Tuna, salmon, or pilchards stirred in. If using pilchards, add an extra helping of tomato ketchup; with the tuna or salmon add a dessertspoon of tartar sauce.

All of the above potato mixes can be combined with the fish, and can be moulded into fish cakes, and stored in fridge or freezer. Lightly fry in a little olive oil.

To make garlic mash, add 2-3 cloves of garlic peeled to the potatoes before boiling, then boil up with the potatoes and mash in.

AUBERGINE BAKE/*EGG PLANT**
1 aubergine/*egg plant**
1 red onion, finely chopped
2 cloves of garlic, finely diced
2 large tomatoes, thinly sliced
1 carrot, peeled

Sun dried tomatoes in olive oil
4 mushrooms, thinly sliced
Salt and pepper
6 oz/170g low fat cheese

METHOD
Slice aubergine/*egg plant** into ¼ inch/7 mm thick slices. Shave peeled carrot into strips with a peeler.
Oil a medium sized roasting tin with olive oil, and place the aubergines/*egg plant** to cover the bottom. Brush with olive oil from the sun dried tomatoes.
Take the sun-dried tomatoes and snip them up and over the top of the aubergines.
Then layer the mushrooms, shaved carrots, onions, garlic, and tomatoes. As you put each layer on, season with salt and pepper to taste.
Put the grated cheese over the top, making sure it covers all of the ingredients.
Place in a preheated oven 200 C/400 F/gas mark 6 for 30-40 mins.

Take out and leave to stand for at least 15 minutes, before serving.
This recipe tastes better warm.

This recipe will serve 4 people if eaten with meat, 2 people if served as a dish on its own. This is an ideal dish for vegetarians.

*USA

***

SNACKS

VEGETABLE CRISPS/*CHIPS**
1 carrot, peeled
1 parsnip, peeled
1 small beetroot (optional), peeled
Extra light olive oil
Water
Juice of ½ lemon

Sea salt

METHOD

On a mandolin, finely slice the carrot, parsnip, and beetroot.

Place water and lemon juice in a big bowl.

Put into the water the sliced carrot and parsnip, not the beetroot (if using).

Soak for 5 minutes.

Fill a large pan a quarter full with the olive oil, and heat until suitable for frying.

Drain the sliced vegetables and pat dry in a tea towel or kitchen paper.

Take a small hand full of the vegetables and place gently in the hot oil, making sure you separate the slices as you put them in the oil.

Cook for no more than a few seconds. They will puff up and change colour.

Take out with a straining spoon.

Place on a plate covered with kitchen paper.

Add another handful of vegetables to the oil, and repeat until all the vegetables have been cooked.

Fry the beetroot last.

When the plate is full of the crisps/*chips**, tip the crisps into a large bowl.

Replace the kitchen paper on the plate when soaked with oil.

When all the crisps/*chips* are in the bowl, grind some sea salt over them, and turn the crisps/*chips* with your hands, gently, to mix the salt in.

Eat hot or cold.

They will not keep for more than a day in an airtight container. They are best eaten fresh.

*USA

HANDY SNACKS

Fruit and nuts

Sunflower seeds, pumpkin seeds and chopped apricot mixed together.

Cereal bars

Fruit

Sultanas

***

CHAPTER FIVE
OPTIONAL MEAL PLANS

BREAKFAST
Tinned fruit or fresh fruit with yoghurt and honey.

LUNCH/TEA
Winter salad with tinned mackerel.

DINNER
Oven baked beans with lamb or beef rissoles.

BREAKFAST
Toasted homemade bread with jam or honey.

LUNCH/TEA
Spinach with low fat cream cheese or Feta cheese.

DINNER
Couscous with salmon.

BREAKFAST
Smoothie.

LUNCH/TEA
Soup.

DINNER
Tagliatelle with chorizo.

BREAKFAST
Porridge.

LUNCH/TEA
Sandwiches made with homemade bread.

DINNER
Chicken with Chunky Chopped Roast Vegetables.

***

CHAPTER SIX
WHAT TO EXPECT – THE ULTIMATE GOAL

You will feel younger and because you body is happy, your energy levels will increase and the weight will disappear.

Your weight loss will not be apparent straight away. Your body has to cleanse from the inside out. It will take about a month before you notice the weight loss.

It appears in the face first, around the chin and jowl area, then the neck. The next place is on the bottom. You will notice your trousers become baggy around your bottom.

Your energy levels and memory improve within a week.

I found during the first month, and so did my friends, that the occasional zit appeared on the face. This is due to the insides being cleansed, and the eating plan beginning to work.

Within a week I noticed how soft the skin on my face felt and in a month the skin on the whole of my body felt silky smooth, and as I don't often use moisturiser on my body, I came to the conclusion that my body was naturally moisturising my skin. I had had flaky and cracking skin since putting on the weight and eating incorrectly.

After two months I found that the weight was reducing quite quickly, and safety pins came in very handy, to hold clothes up around my waist, as this was the next place on my body to really lose noticeable weight, even though the rest of my body was losing it as well. I also noticed my watch was loose around my wrist, and I had to push it up my arm. So I thought I would try my ankle bracelet on, and guess what, I could put it on without having to undo the clasp. My shoes didn't fit either, as my feet had lost weight too.

After three months, my stomach was certainly flatter and I could touch my toes, again.

Whilst you are losing your weight, don't go mad buying clothes and shoes, buy just a few clothes and shoes to take yourself through to the next season, because by the next season those clothes will be too big.

Keep on the eating plan and your body will stop at its natural weight. We cannot all be skinny sticks, so don't aim for the impossible.

It took my body a year to shed 6 ½ stone/*91 lbs**. I am now where I want to be with my weight, 10 stone/*140 lbs**, and I feel great.

If you have more than 6 ½ stone/*91 lbs** to lose, your body could lose it faster, because you are now looking after it and nourishing it. When you become more active, the weight reduces quicker. I know that being over weight, exercise is not easy to do, as you get breathless quickly and your joints ache, but by following the eating plan the weight starts to go, which means you can then start with gentle exercise. I found walking the easiest and cheapest, also you can explore your own neighbourhood whilst walking and meet new people. Don't try and walk at a fast pace at first, just walk at a speed comfortable to you, and as far as you feel able to do. Each time you go for a walk go a little further and go a little faster, remember your body has to get used to this funny thing called exercise, and it is like learning to walk all over again. Enjoy the walk don't make it a chore and walk at a comfortable speed; you are doing it for pleasure not a marathon.

At the beginning of the eating plan, you might crave for those banned foods, that you had taught you mind and body to expect. Be strong, and say **NO** to them. As I have said before, once your body is re educated, those banned foods will taste awful, and say to yourself, "I AM ALLERGIC TO FAT, CHEMICALS, PRESERVATIVES AND ADDITIVES. I AM NOT DESIGNED TO EAT THESE".

Remember if you go out to eat, choose what to eat wisely, drink your apple juice afterwards, to counteract any fat content, chemicals, and preservatives.

This eating plan is not made to spoil your fun, it is for making you healthy, to live longer and to have more fun, with all your new gained energy.

Turn back the clock and go forward again.

Enjoy eating yourself thin, like I did, I now feel great and bounding with energy.

*USA